The Glycemic Load Counter

The Glycemic Load Counter

A Pocket Guide to GL and GI Values for Over 800 Foods

Dr. Mabel Blades

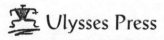 Ulysses Press

Published in the U.S. by
ULYSSES PRESS
P.O. Box 3440
Berkeley, CA 94703
www.ulyssespress.com

First published as *The GI Counter* in Great Britain in 2007
by Kyle Cathie Limited

ISBN10: 1-56975-664-3
ISBN13: 978-1-56975-664-5
Library of Congress Control Number: 2007907766

Printed in Canada by Webcom

10 9 8 7 6 5 4 3 2

Editorial and production: Nick Denton-Brown, Lauren Harrison,
    Tamara Kowalski
Cover design: Double R Design
Interior design and production: whatIdesign @ whatweb.com

Distributed by Publishers Group West

NOTE TO READERS
This book has been written and published strictly for informational and educational purposes only. It is not intended to serve as medical advice or to be any form of medical treatment. You should always consult your physician before altering or changing any aspect of your medical treatment and/or undertaking a diet regimen, including the GL guidelines as described in this book. Do not stop or change any prescription medications without the guidance and advice of your physician. Any use of the information in this book is made on the reader's good judgment after consulting with his or her physician and is the reader's sole responsibility. This book is not intended to diagnose or treat any medical condition and is not a substitute for a physician.

TABLE OF CONTENTS

Introduction

The Glycemic Index and Glycemic Load are values given to different carbohydrate foods based on how they impact blood sugar levels. The GL is a development of the Glycemic Index that takes into account the amount of carbohydrates in a food and the body's response to them.

There are many reasons why you might want to keep an eye on your GL intake, and this counter was developed to help you choose foods wisely rather than having to look at lots of other lists, websites and packages. And because carbohydrate content or GL should not be considered in isolation, I have also provided information on calorie content and fat levels.

So What Exactly is GI?

The Glycemic Index measures the way in which we break down carbohydrate foods into the simple sugar glucose, which is then absorbed and used in our bodies for energy. Like the GI, the Glycemic Load is an index that ranks foods according to their effect on blood sugar. The difference, however, is that GI gives us information on how quickly blood sugar rises after we eat 50g (about 2oz) of digestible carbohydrates in various foods—which is nearly impossible to do in some cases. You'd have to eat two pounds of watermelon to get 50g of digestible carbohydrates out of it! The GL, on the other hand, reflects the change in blood sugar caused by eating a normal portion of food. It's a more accurate assessment of foods because it reflects the amount of carbohydrates you actually eat. Watermelon, as mentioned before, is a great example of this. It has a high GI (about 70) because the carbohydrate it contains is glucose, which is pure sugar. But because watermelon contains very little glucose overall, it has a low GL of just 5 for a normal-sized serving. You would have to eat ten times a normal portion of watermelon to get the same rise in blood sugar as you would from eating a normal serving of white bread (which, under the confusing Glycemic Index system has an almost identical GI as watermelon). So whereas GI would have you think that watermelon is bad for you, GL proves that it's actually great!

Why is a Low-GI Diet Good for You?

Foods with a low GL sustain our blood sugar levels, or rather blood glucose levels, for longer than those with a high GL, which cause a peak in blood sugar levels followed by a slump. When our blood sugars are maintained at a moderate level, we tend not to feel hungry. When the level zooms up after eating a high GL food, the dramatic dip that follows takes blood sugars down to a level at which we can feel really hungry. It must be emphasized that the GL is concerned solely with carbohydrates, so proteins and fats all have zero GL because they are not made up of glucose units. This fact has led to some controversy about the value of a low-GL diet. But in my experience, most people who are trying to lose weight, or are keeping an eye on their diet for specific health reasons, are sensible enough to know that fats are high in calories and that too many lead to weight gain!

What are the Ranges for GL?

- Low-GL foods are those with a value below 10

- Medium-GL foods are those foods with value of 11–19

- High-GL foods are those with a value of 20+

GL & Weight Loss

The value of the GL is to help you make more prudent choices regarding foods. In general, a woman wanting to lose weight on 1500 calories per day should eat about

200g of carbohydrates, and a man trying to lose weight on 2000 calories per day, about 260g. At least half of this should have a low GL (below 10). This will result in a slow but steady weight loss of about one to two pounds per week.

The main point is to try and keep mostly to low-GL carbohydrate foods. That means eating lots of fresh foods like fruits and vegetables, which we all know are the basis of a healthy diet. It is also sensible to combine carbohydrate foods with a protein food such as fish, eggs or cheese, or vegetable sources of protein like nuts. For flavor and ease in cooking, perhaps add a little healthy fat like olive oil or canola oil. Foods such as meat, fish, cheese and eggs all have a GL of zero, but they do contain different amounts of fat and provide a source of calories. So it is important to take a common sense approach and not to base the diet on these foods alone.

Although many people are obsessed with their weight and trying to lose it, they really should be trying to lose body fat while preserving muscle tissue. This means exercise has to be included in their daily patterns.

This type of low-GL diet makes a sensible, balanced eating program, which will keep you feeling full and energetic, while providing all the healthy nutrients your body needs.

Conditions Helped by a Low-GL Diet

A diet with a low GL is considered to be helpful for a number of conditions, including:

- *Managing weight loss and preventing weight gain* by promoting a feeling of fullness and avoiding very low blood sugar levels, which send you running for a snack.
- *Diabetes,* because it helps stabilize blood sugar levels.
- *Raised cholesterol levels,* because the soluble fibers found in such low-GL foods such as oats, fruits and vegetables reduce the absorption of saturated fat and cholesterol.
- *Polycystic ovary syndrome (PCOS),* from which increasing numbers of women (some say as many as 10%–15%) suffer and in which maintenance of blood sugar is important. Symptoms of PCOS include irregular or absent periods, very greasy skin, facial hair growth, hair loss, mood swings and difficulties with excessive weight gain.
- *Metabolic syndrome* (sometimes referred to as syndrome X), which is the precondition for Type 2 diabetes and coronary heart disease. It is characterized by weight gain (especially around the middle area, creating the so-called "apple shape"), raised blood pressure, high blood sugar and high cholesterol levels, as well as raised triglyceride levels
- *Raised triglyceride levels*, which can contribute to coronary heart disease in a similar way to raised cholesterol levels.
- *Improving behavior in young people*, due to the sustained energy levels that help concentration and good behavior.
- *Digestive problems such as irritable bowel syndrome*, because the diet includes more fiber and promotes a healthy bacterial population in the digestive tract.

- *Constipation*, which is often due to too little fiber and fluids in the diet. Although people tend not to talk about this, it is both common and unpleasant. A low-GL diet, with its generous amounts of vegetables and fruits (and therefore fiber), as well as plenty of fluids, can be of great assistance in relieving the problem.
- *Low blood sugar levels (hypoglycemia)* can be helped by the sustained blood sugar levels from frequent snacks of low-GL foods.

How is the GL Calculated?

The GL is calculated by multiplying the amount of carbohydrates in a normal sized portion of the food by the GI of the food, and then dividing by 100.

So, for example, baked beans in tomato sauce have an average GI of 48, which counts as low. An average 100g portion contains 15g of carbohydrate, so the GL is 48 x 15 = 720, divided by 100, thus the GL is 7, which is also low.

However, this means doing a fairly complicated calculation for each food, whereas the GI exists as an established measure. It's one of those areas where using your common sense and taking calorie count and portion size into account will take you a long way.

What is a Portion?

Knowing portion sizes is a sensible way to avoid taking in excess calories and fat. As a rough guide (remember this is not an exact science!), a portion is:

- A medium-sized apple, peach, banana or pear
- Half a large fruit such as a grapefruit
- 2 plums
- A slice of melon, mango or pineapple
- A handful of berries or grapes
- 3 tablespoons of canned or stewed fruit
- Dried fruit also counts; a portion is about the same amount as if the fruit were fresh. For example, three dried apricots, two dried figs or a handful of raisins.
- A small glass or carton of fruit juice. This only counts as one portion per day no matter how much you drink because the fiber is removed in the process of making juice.
- A cereal bowlful of salad
- 3 tablespoons of cooked vegetables
- A handful of raw vegetable sticks
- 100–150g raw weight of meat, poultry or fish. This means a piece about the size of a pack of cards.
- 25–30g of cheese. Around the size of a matchbox, which looks like a lot and goes even further if it is grated.
- 2 medium eggs
- A small handful of nuts and seeds

This book considers a portion size to be 100g, or about 4oz. This portion allows people to adjust the diet to their own lifestyle and eating patterns. Where foods like herbs and spices are listed, the GL is counted as zero because you are very unlikely to eat 100g of those. That means you can have flavorful and spicy meals without concern for their GL value.

Where information is available, values for the same food may vary from one list to another because of different varieties of fruits, vegetables or products. For the purposes of this book, common values have been taken and some estimates have been made based on averages.

What are Carbohydrate Foods?

Carbohydrate foods are the source of energy that all cells of our body can easily use. They are also the only source of energy for our brains. They are a less concentrated source of energy than fats, alcohol or protein. This means that we can eat more of them to get the same amount of calories, which is good news for those with big appetites.

There are two main types of carbohydrates—sugars and starches. The sugary carbohydrates are those foods that contain a lot of sugar, such as jam, cakes, cookies, candy, chocolate and many soft drinks. Starchy foods contain a large proportion of starch and include bread, pasta, rice, potatoes, breakfast cereals and noodles. During the process of digestion and absorption, both sugars and starches are broken down into the tiny molecules of sugars of which they are composed. It is this sugar that is absorbed into the bloodstream.

However, carbohydrate foods are not made up exclusively of carbohydrates. They may well contain other nutrients such as protein, fiber, vitamins, minerals and fat, as well as water. For example, white bread—classified as a "carbohydrate food"—consists of approximately 46% carbohydrate, 8% protein, 2% fiber, 2% fat and 39% water, and the rest of it is made up of minerals like calcium, iron, zinc and sodium and the B vitamin group.

The predominant sugar that circulates in our blood is the simple sugar glucose. It is derived mainly from starchy carbohydrates such as bread, pasta, breakfast cereals, rice, potatoes, couscous, cookies and crackers. "Complex" sugars such as table sugar (sucrose) also have a component of glucose, as does the sugar in milk (lactose) and malt, which is used in flavorings for foods such as breakfast cereals. Various factors affect the GL of a carbohydrate food. These include:

- *The way the food is prepared.* For example, fruit juice has a higher GL than whole fruit, because in making it you lose the fiber that slows down the absorption of glucose. Another good reason for eating plenty of fresh fruit.
- *The structure of the starch and sugars.* Different varieties of the same food may contain different types of starch, so they may have a different GL. Some plant breeders are working on food crops such as potatoes and rice to produce varieties with a lower GL.

- *Tough fibrous coatings like those found in seeds.* These have to be broken down during digestion, which means they take more time to be attacked in the digestive process and thus they have a low GL.

- *Soluble fibers* like those found in oats, lentils and barley. These slow down digestion, giving these foods a low GL.

- *Reheating.* With some carbohydrate foods this can change the structure of the starch, which is why canned potatoes (bought pre-cooked and then reheated), have a lower GL than ordinary boiled ones. Freshly cooked foods retain more of their vitamins.

- *Mixing low-GL carbohydrate foods with those with a higher GL.* Combining foods with different values in a meal or snack lowers the overall GL of the mixture.

- *Adding foods that contain zero GL.* Adding these foods, such as fat or protein, will reduce the overall GL of a meal (but be careful about eating too much fat).

Calories from Nutrients

All foods and beverages (with the exception of water) provide energy in the form of calories.

- Carbohydrates provide 3.75 calories per gram

- Protein provides 4 calories per gram

- Fat provides 9 calories per gram

- Alcohol provides 7 calories per gram

To lose weight we need to burn more calories than we take in, which means reducing the overall calorie content of the food we eat and increasing activity so that the body uses up its stores of fat.

Carbohydrates

Watching carbohydrate intake is particularly important for those with diabetes, but may also be sensible for some women with polycystic ovary syndrome (PCOS). People of either sex who have raised triglycerides (a sticky substance, which can be found in the blood and which can clog up the arteries in a way similar to the harmful type of cholesterol) may also be advised to limit the amount of sugary carbohydrates that they eat.

Fruits and Vegetables

We should eat at least five portions of fruits and vegetables each day. This is about 400g in total. (Remember that potatoes are classified as a starchy food and do not count towards the five portions.) Not only are fruit and vegetables generally low in calories, but they also contain those all-important protective substances of antioxidants and fiber.

Fats

Although fats have a GL of zero because they contain no carbohydrates, they are higher in calories than carbohydrates, protein and even alcohol. For many people, reducing the amount of fat in their diet reduces overall calorie intake and helps with weight loss.

We all need some fat in our diet for maintenance of the brain and nervous tissues and as a base for making some hormones and vitamins. Monounsaturates such as olive oil and canola oil are considered to be good fats. Polyunsaturates, found in soy oil and corn oil are also considered to be beneficial. Omega-3 fatty acids are essential for brain development and function as well as general health, because they are associated with lower levels of coronary heart disease. They are found mainly in oily fish (see page 23).

Excess fat, particularly of the saturated type found in animal products such as lard, whole milk, cheese, butter and the fat on meat is also linked with coronary heart disease. Knowing the fat content of foods can assist those with this problem as well as those who are watching their fat intake for other reasons. Saturated fat is also found in foods such as pastries, cakes, creamy sauces, margarine, coconut cream and coconut oil. (Beware of these last two—many people are amazed by how much saturated fat there is in dishes such as Thai-style curries, which use these ingredients.)

Alcohol
The USDA recommends that alcohol be consumed sensibly and in moderation. This is defined as up to one drink a day for a woman and up to two drinks a day for a man.

Fiber
Dietary fiber used to be known as "roughage" and is scientifically known as non-starch polysaccharide ANSI.

It is found only in plant foods such as cereals, fruits and vegetables. The body cannot use it for energy, so in humans its purpose is to add bulk to the diet. It is, however, the main source of energy for animals like sheep and cows.

There are two types of fiber. Soluble fiber is found mainly in oats, barley, fruits and vegetables—especially dried vegetables such as lentils, split peas and beans. Insoluble fiber is found mainly in wheat products such as bread, pasta and breakfast cereals. Soluble fiber is important in moderating blood cholesterol and blood sugar levels, while insoluble fiber is particularly beneficial for bowel health. Both types are filling, so eating plenty of foods containing fiber, especially fruits and vegetables, really helps to fill you up.

Sodium
The chemical name for salt is sodium chloride, and sodium is the damaging component found in it. Anyone with high blood pressure or heart problems is likely to be advised by their doctor to limit their sodium intake, but today we are all encouraged to reduce the amount of salt we eat.

Other Nutritional Information
To help you make choices on how to fit a low-GL diet into other aspects of a healthy lifestyle, this book provides calorie counts and information on the fat and carbohydrate content of foods. Remember that the values of these nutrients can vary with different brands from different manufacturers, so

if you are comparing package information, you may see some slight discrepancies.

Remember that losing weight should always be done slowly, no more than one to two pounds a week if you expect to keep the weight off. Indeed, what you really should be trying to do is lose body fat and acquire more lean body mass as you get fitter and develop more muscles. If you are severely overweight or are gaining weight, it may be worth trying to maintain it for a week by eating sensibly, choosing plenty of low-GL carbohydrates, as well as doing more exercise such as walking. If you do not manage to control your eating habits and stop gaining weight, it is unlikely that you will be able to stick to a weight-loss eating pattern and maintain a new lower weight. In this case, you may be advised to consult your doctor for further assistance and perhaps a referral to a registered dietitian.

The following are easy tips for making healthier choices:

- Base your meals on starchy foods
- Eat lots of fruit and vegetables
- Eat more fish, including a portion of oily fish each week
- Cut down on saturated fat and sugar
- Try to eat less salt—no more than 6g a day for adults
- Get active and try to be a healthy weight
- Drink plenty of water
- Don't skip breakfast

Base your meals on starchy foods

These foods should make up about a third of your daily intake. Starchy foods are major sources of energy, B vitamins and dietary fiber.

This is easy to achieve on a low-GL diet—it just means a few substitutions. For example, use thick slices of whole grain, seeded bread or grain breads instead of white, brown or whole-wheat in your sandwiches. These breads also make delicious toast and great bread puddings.

Use small potatoes boiled in their skins instead of mashed or peeled, boiled potatoes, or serve boiled potatoes with a low-GL food such as baked beans to reduce the overall GL level.

Swap white rice for brown basmati, which has the lowest GL of any rice, and include more pasta dishes on your menu.

Try adding low-GL items like barley to your soup, or experiment with bulgur wheat in casseroles or as an alternative to rice or potatoes.

Eat lots of fruit and vegetables

In general, we are still not eating those all important five portions of fruit and vegetables each day.

A low-GL diet really encourages the inclusion of more vegetables. Since most vegetables have a low GL, they reduce the overall GL of a meal. Vegetables are also low in fat, low in salt and low in calories—all good reasons to eat plenty of them!

Fresh vegetables have more flavor, especially when they're freshly picked from the garden. But these days a range of frozen, canned and "ready-to-steam" vegetables is available too, so there is no excuse for not including them. While canned and dried vegetables will have lost vitamins during their processing, frozen ones have the vitamins safely locked in so are probably the best alternative to fresh. If you choose canned vegetables, look at the sodium content and go for those without added salt.

Using a steamer or microwave in which vegetables can be cooked in minutes is the best way to preserve flavor and color. Vegetables can also be added to a casserole in a slow cooker, which brings out their full flavor.

Many fruits, especially apples, bananas, cherries, plums and berries, also have a low GL. They make excellent snacks and additions to cereals, and bananas are great in sandwiches. Fruit is also the perfect accompaniment to ice creams and yogurts. And, like vegetables, it is generally low in calories, fat and sodium.

Having been deeply immersed in looking at information on nutrition and GL in the course of preparing this book, if there is one thing I want to emphasize, it is to eat more vegetables. They contain many protective nutrients, are low in calories and fat, have wonderful flavor and are generally inexpensive.

Eat more fish, including a portion of oily fish each week

Fish, like all protein food, has a GL of zero, so it pairs well with high-GL foods. Avoid frying it, especially in batter or bread crumbs, to keep the fat content down.

Salmon, mackerel, trout, herring, fresh tuna, sardines and eel are all classified as oily fish, and therefore are good sources of Omega-3 fatty acids. They can be combined with potatoes or pasta and vegetables in various hot dishes, or eaten hot or cold with salad.

Cut down on saturated fat and sugar

Cutting down on saturated fat is associated with promoting heart health. When looking at the fat content figures given in this book, bear in mind that 20g or more of fat per 100g in a food is generally considered "a lot" and 3g or less is "a little." A lot of saturated fat is 5g per 100g of food and a little is 1g per 100g. Sugar is associated with dental decay when eaten too frequently. 10g of sugar per 100g of food represents high sugar content and 2g per 100g is low.

Try to eat less salt—no more than 6g a day for adults

Most of our salt intake comes from manufactured foods and because a low-GL diet is based on lots of fresh foods like vegetables and fruits, it should be relatively easy to keep below the 6g guideline.

When it comes to salt, 2.5g of salt or 0.5g of sodium per 100g of food is regarded as a lot. A low level of salt is 0.25g of salt or 0.1g of sodium per 100g of food.

Ready-made foods are often higher in salt than the homemade equivalent, so this is another good reason to emphasize home-cooked dishes.

Some stock or bouillon cubes, often used for flavor, are high in salt. Use them sparingly, or instead experiment with a range of different herbs and spices, many of which have strong and distinct flavors. This means you can reduce the amount of salt you add to food.

Get active and try to be a healthy weight

Many people find that sticking to a low-GL diet is an excellent and satisfying way to lose weight. The only guaranteed way to lose weight (and body fat) is to use up more energy, or calories, than you consume. So the calorie counts provided in this book will help you to calculate how many you are taking in. Remember to aim at losing only one to two pounds per week.

Becoming more active by including activities like walking in daily life will burn up some of the calories, and you're more likely to stick with it than a gym membership.

Drink plenty of water

We all need over a liter of water each day as part of the recommended total intake of two liters of fluid. Water is calorie free and zero GL, so you can and should drink a lot of it. All types of water are good for hydration and increasingly there is a trend away from bottled water toward fresh, chilled tap water.

Sugary drinks provide extra calories, as does alcohol, which can also be damaging to the liver if consumed in excess.

Teas and coffees contain caffeine, and while excessive amounts are harmful, normal quantities (3–4 cups a day) add to that all-important fluid intake. Try to use skim or low-fat milk and avoid adding sugar. If you have a weakness for lattes, remember that many are made with whole milk.

Don't skip breakfast
This is one of the most important meals of the day, and is very easy to have in the form of a low-GL food like oatmeal. Without breakfast, our blood sugar can slump midmorning, which makes us more likely to succumb to the temptation of a high-calorie snack like candy or cookies for an instant energy boost. It is no wonder that breakfast-eaters tend to be slimmer! If you have to get up at the crack of dawn and rush for a train, then have something like fruit or a low-GL cereal when you get to work.

How Foods are Listed
Foods included in this book are divided into categories such as fruit, vegetables and dairy products. Because people think of different foods in different ways, a few items have been listed twice. For example, potatoes are grouped with starchy carbohydrate foods like bread, pasta and rice. However, many people think of them as vegetables and this is where they are found in the supermarket. So for ease of use, potatoes are listed on their own. Similarly, butter is

considered a fat, but many people consider it a dairy food, so it is listed in both sections.

A few reminders on using these tables:

- Low-GL foods are those with a GL below 10, medium are those between 11 and 19, and high are those with a GL of 20 and above.

- GL may differ from brand to brand of the same food, so use these figures as a guide rather than as absolute values.

- Information on the energy content of food is given in calories per 100g.

- Carbohydrate content and fat levels are also given per 100g.

- If you are a woman trying to lose weight, aim for getting 1500 calories a day; if you are a man, 2000 calories each day.

- A healthy diet includes less than 70g per day of fat if you are a woman and less than 85g if you are a man.

Finally

This GL counter aims to help you to eat a healthy low-GL diet. Do not be obsessive about it, but use it for guidance, and remember that there are no bad foods, but there are unbalanced and bad diets!

Chapter One

Breads, Pastries, Pastas and Grains

Carbohydrates can be diet disasters because they tend to have high-GL scores that send your blood sugar levels soaring. But there are many lower-GL alternatives that keep you feeling fuller longer because your blood sugar stays at a normal level. Choose breads, pastas and breakfast cereals made with whole grains rather than white flour so they metabolize slower.

	GL	GI	Calories	Carbs	Fat
BAGEL					
white	**42**	72	273	57.8	1.8
BAGUETTE					
plain	**53**	95	263	56.1	1.9
BARLEY					
pearl	**7**	25	120	27.6	0.6
BREAD					
brown	**31**	73	207	42.1	2.0
fruit	**18**	47	187	38.9	2.6
gluten-free	**76**	78	258	98.0	12.0
oat	**20**	47	237	43.5	3.0
rye, no grains	**23**	51	219	45.8	1.7
rye, with grains	**19**	41	219	45.8	1.7
sourdough rye	**20**	53	184	37.0	1.2
soy & flaxseed	**12**	41	252	29.8	10.1
stuffing	**14**	74	97	19.3	1.5
sunflower	**23**	57	240	39.6	4.7
sunflower & barley	**23**	57	240	39.9	6.1
white	**34**	70	235	49.3	1.9
white, added fiber	**34**	68	230	49.6	1.5

	GL	GI	Calories	Carbs	Fat
BREAD (CONTINUED)					
white, spelt flour	**36**	74	235	49.3	1.9
whole-wheat	**32**	77	217	42.0	2.9

BREAKFAST CEREALS

	GL	GI	Calories	Carbs	Fat
All-Bran	**15**	30	270	48.5	3.5
bite-size, whole grain	**54**	71	411	76.1	9.8
Bran Buds	**30**	58	273	52.0	2.9
bran cereal, noodle-shaped	**15**	34	270	44.0	1.8
Bran Flakes	**53**	74	330	71.2	1.9
Cheerios	**60**	74	368	80.7	3.8
Cocoa Krispies	**70**	77	383	91.5	2.5
Cornflakes	**69**	77	376	89.6	0.7
Frosted Flakes	**52**	55	381	94.6	0.6
Grape Nuts	**14**	71	345	20.0	2.0
muesli, Swiss	**40**	56	363	72.2	6.7
oat bran	**27**	55	345	49.7	9.7
oatmeal, instant, low-fat milk	**9**	66	100	13.8	2.8
oatmeal, made with water	**3**	42	46	8.1	1.1
Puffed Wheat	**54**	80	321	67.3	1.3
Raisin Bran	**44**	61	332	71.5	1.5
Rice Krispies	**76**	82	382	92.9	1.0

	GL	GI	Calories	Carbs	Fat
BREAKFAST CEREALS (CONTINUED)					
Shredded Wheat	**54**	75	332	71.7	2.2
Special K	**41**	54	373	75.0	1.0
Wheaties	**52**	69	352	75.5	2.0
whole-grain cereal cluster	**44**	66	351	66.0	9.0
BUCKWHEAT					
boiled	**46**	54	364	84.9	1.5
CAKE					
angel food	**37**	67	380	55.0	15.5
banana	**24**	51	257	46.9	7.4
carrot	**29**	62	341	47.3	16.3
fruit	**31**	54	371	57.9	14.8
sponge	**24**	46	467	52.4	27.2
vanilla-iced	**22**	42	490	52.4	30.6
COUSCOUS					
boiled	**33**	65	227	51.3	1.0
CROISSANT					
plain	**29**	67	373	43.3	26.0

	GL	GI	Calories	Carbs	Fat
CUPCAKE					
plain	**39**	73	468	54.0	24.0
DOUGHNUT					
plain	**37**	76	336	48.8	14.5
ENGLISH MUFFIN					
plain	**27**	69	177	38.6	0.9
FLAN					
baked	**43**	65	320	65.7	4.5
GNOCCHI					
boiled	**23**	68	152	33.6	0.3
HAMBURGER BUN					
plain	**30**	61	264	48.8	5.0
MUFFINS					
blueberry	**25**	59	355	42.7	18.2
chocolate chip	**28**	53	385	52.3	18.2

	GL	GI	Calories	Carbs	Fat
PANCAKES					
from scratch	**23**	67	302	34.9	16.3
from mix	**18**	67	152	27.4	1.8
PASTA					
egg noodles, boiled	**7**	57	62	13.0	0.5
egg noodles, fried	**5**	46	147	11.3	11.5
fettucine	**19**	40	264	47.4	2.9
linguine	**16**	52	150	30.1	0.7
macaroni	**9**	47	86	18.5	0.5
ravioli, meat-filled	**3**	39	75	7.0	0.5
spaghetti, brown	**9**	37	113	23.2	0.9
spaghetti, white	**8**	38	104	22.2	0.7
spiral-shaped	**8**	43	86	18.5	0.1
tortellini, cheese	**13**	50	183	25.5	5.1
vermicelli	**12**	35	160	32.9	0.8
PASTRY					
plain	**28**	59	451	46.8	28.1
PITA					
white	**31**	57	255	55.1	1.3

	GL	GI	Calories	Carbs	Fat

POP TART

plain	48	70	386	69.0	10.0

PRETZELS

plain	66	83	381	79.2	3.5

QUINOA

boiled	29	53	309	55.7	5.0

RICE

long grain & wild	18	58	138	30.9	1.3
arborio	21	69	138	30.9	1.3
basmati, boiled	18	58	138	30.9	1.3
basmati, microwaved	13	52	116	24.9	1.2
brown	22	70	141	32.1	1.1
long grain, boiled	17	56	138	30.9	1.3
long grain, microwaved	13	52	110	24.9	1.2
white	30	98	138	30.9	1.3

SCONE

plain	49	92	364	53.7	14.8

	GL	GI	Calories	Carbs	Fat
TACO SHELL					
corn	**41**	68	506	61.0	23.0
TAPIOCA PUDDING					
plain	**10**	81	75	12.4	1.8
WAFFLES					
plain	**30**	76	334	39.6	16.7

Chapter Two

Meats, Chicken, Seafood and Eggs

Proteins like beef, chicken, fish and eggs contain no carbohydrates, so they tend to have a GL score of zero. But be careful—they can be high in fat and calories. If you choose lean meats and try to incorporate more seafood into your diet, you'll get lots of good proteins, minerals and flavors without sacrificing your waistline.

	GL	GI	Calories	Carbs	Fat
ANCHOVIES					
canned, in oil	**0**	0	191	0.0	10.0
BACON					
fried	**0**	0	350	0.0	28.5
grilled	**0**	0	337	0.0	26.9
raw	**0**	0	276	0.0	23.6
BASS					
raw	**0**	0	100	0.0	2.5
BEEF					
brisket, lean, boiled	**0**	0	225	0.0	11.0
brisket, lean, raw	**0**	0	139	0.0	6.1
brisket, boiled	**0**	0	268	0.0	17.4
brisket, raw	**0**	0	218	0.0	16.0
burgers, fried	**0**	0	329	0.1	23.9
burgers, grilled	**0**	0	326	0.1	24.4
burgers, raw	**0**	0	291	0.1	24.7
corned, canned	**0**	0	205	1.0	10.9
corned, raw	**0**	0	119	0.0	0.4
corned, raw, dried	**0**	0	250	0.0	1.5
flank steak, lean, braised	**0**	0	225	0.0	9.7

	GL	GI	Calories	Carbs	Fat
BEEF (CONTINUED)					
flank steak, lean, raw	0	0	139	0.0	5.7
flank steak, lean, slow-cooked	0	0	197	0.0	7.9
flank steak, braised	0	0	246	0.0	12.7
flank steak, raw	0	0	160	0.0	8.6
flank steak, slow-cooked	0	0	217	0.0	11.2
flank, lean, pot roast	0	0	253	0.0	14.0
flank, lean, raw	0	0	175	0.0	9.3
flank, raw	0	0	266	0.0	20.8
flank, pot roast	0	0	309	0.0	22.3
ground, extra-lean, raw	0	0	174	0.0	9.6
ground, extra-lean, stewed	0	0	177	0.0	8.7
ground, microwaved	0	0	263	0.0	17.5
ground, stewed	0	0	209	0.0	13.6
ribs, lean, microwaved	0	0	243	0.0	11.4
ribs, lean, roast	0	0	236	0.0	11.4
ribs, microwaved	0	0	300	0.0	20.4
ribs, raw	0	0	253	0.0	19.8
ribs, roast	0	0	306	0.0	20.5
round, medium-rare	0	0	222	0.0	11.4
round, raw, lean & fat	0	0	198	0.0	12.9
round, well-done	0	0	244	0.0	12.5

MEATS, CHICKEN, SEAFOOD AND EGGS

	GL	GI	Calories	Carbs	Fat
BEEF (CONTINUED)					
rump roast, lean, pot roast	0	0	193	0.0	6.3
rump roast, lean, raw	0	0	134	0.0	4.3
rump roast, lean, salted, boiled	0	0	184	0.0	6.9
short loin, lean, raw	0	0	135	0.0	4.5
short loin, lean, roast	0	0	188	0.0	6.5
short loin, roast	0	0	233	0.0	12.6
short loin, raw, lean & fat	0	0	201	0.0	12.7
sirloin, fried, lean	0	0	183	0.0	6.6
sirloin, grilled, lean	0	0	177	0.0	5.9
sirloin, raw, lean & fat	0	0	174	0.0	10.1
steak, fried	0	0	302	0.5	22.2
steak, grilled	0	0	305	0.5	23.9
steak, raw	0	0	285	0.2	22.2
steak, slow-cooked	0	0	197	0.0	7.9
stewing steak, lean, pressure-cooked	0	0	199	0.0	6.5
stewing steak, lean, raw	0	0	122	0.0	3.5
stewing steak, lean, stewed	0	0	185	0.0	6.3
BREAM					
raw	0	0	96	0.0	2.9

	GL	GI	Calories	Carbs	Fat

CANADIAN BACON

	GL	GI	Calories	Carbs	Fat
crispy, grilled	0	0	313	0.0	18.8
dry-cured, fried	0	0	295	0.0	22.0
fat-trimmed, grilled	0	0	214	0.0	12.3
fat-trimmed, raw	0	0	136	0.0	6.7
grilled	0	0	287	0.0	21.6
microwaved	0	0	307	0.0	23.3
raw	0	0	136	0.0	6.7
reduced-salt, grilled	0	0	282	0.0	20.6
smoked, grilled	0	0	293	0.0	22.1

CATFISH

	GL	GI	Calories	Carbs	Fat
raw	0	0	96	0.0	2.8
steamed	0	0	119	0.0	3.7

CHICKEN

	GL	GI	Calories	Carbs	Fat
breast, grilled, no skin	0	0	148	0.0	2.2
dark meat, raw	0	0	109	0.0	2.8
drumsticks, roasted	0	0	185	0.0	9.1
leg quarter, meat & skin, baked	0	0	217	0.0	13.9
leg quarter, meat & skin, raw	0	0	193	0.0	13.3
leg quarter, meat & skin, roast	0	0	236	0.0	16.9
leg quarter, meat only, baked	0	0	176	0.0	8.4

	GL	GI	Calories	Carbs	Fat
CHICKEN (CONTINUED)					
meat & skin	**0**	0	230	0.0	17.7
nuggets	**9**	46	265	19.5	13.0
strips, stir-fried	**0**	0	161	0.0	4.6
white meat, raw	**0**	0	106	0.0	1.1
wing quarter, baked	**0**	0	164	0.0	6.3
wing quarter, meat & skin, baked	**0**	0	210	0.0	12.5
wing quarter, meat & skin, raw	**0**	0	193	0.0	12.4
wing quarter, meat & skin, roast	**0**	0	226	0.0	14.1
CLAMS					
canned, in brine	**0**	0	77	1.9	0.6
COD					
dried & salted, boiled	**0**	0	138	0.0	0.9
dried & salted, raw	**0**	0	130	0.0	0.7
fillet, baked	**0**	0	96	trace	1.2
fillet, grilled	**0**	0	80	trace	1.3
fillet, poached	**0**	0	94	trace	1.1
fillet, raw	**0**	0	80	0.0	0.7
smoked, poached	**0**	0	101	trace	1.6
smoked, raw	**0**	0	79	0.0	0.6
steamed	**0**	0	83	0.0	0.9

	GL	GI	Calories	Carbs	Fat

CORNISH GAME HEN

| raw | 0 | 0 | 202 | 0.0 | 13.9 |

CRAB

| canned, in brine | 0 | 0 | 77 | 0.0 | 0.5 |
| meat, boiled | 0 | 0 | 128 | 0.0 | 5.5 |

DUCK

crispy, Chinese	0	0	331	0.3	24.2
meat & skin, roasted	0	0	388	0.0	49.6
meat only, raw	0	0	137	0.0	6.5
meat only, roasted	0	0	195	0.0	10.4

EEL

| jellied | 0 | 0 | 98 | trace | 7.1 |
| raw | 0 | 0 | 168 | 0.0 | 11.3 |

EGG

boiled	0	0	147	trace	10.8
chicken, raw	0	0	151	trace	11.1
custard	4	35	118	11.0	6.0
duck, raw	0	0	163	trace	11.8
fried	0	0	179	trace	13.9

	GL	GI	Calories	Carbs	Fat
EGG (CONTINUED)					
poached	0	0	147	trace	10.8
scrambled	0	0	160	trace	11.6
white, raw	0	0	36	trace	trace
FISH STICKS					
oven-baked	6	38	200	16.6	8.9
raw	5	38	171	14.2	7.8
FLOUNDER					
raw	0	0	74	0.0	1.2
GOOSE					
roasted, meat & skin	0	0	301	0.0	21.2
HADDOCK					
grilled	0	0	104	0.0	0.8
raw	0	0	81	0.0	0.6
smoked, raw	0	0	81	0.0	0.6
smoked, steamed	0	0	101	0.0	0.9
steamed	0	0	89	0.0	0.6

	GL	GI	Calories	Carbs	Fat
HAKE					
grilled	**0**	0	113	0.0	2.7
raw	**0**	0	92	0.0	2.2
HALIBUT					
grilled	**0**	0	121	0.0	2.2
raw	**0**	0	103	0.0	1.9
steamed	**0**	0	131	0.0	4.0
HAM					
baked	**0**	0	107	1.0	3.3
HERRING					
dried & salted	**0**	0	168	0.0	7.4
fried	**0**	0	204	1.0	15.1
grilled	**0**	0	181	0.0	11.2
pickled	**0**	0	209	10.0	11.1
raw	**0**	0	190	0.0	13.2

MEATS, CHICKEN, SEAFOOD AND EGGS

	GL	GI	Calories	Carbs	Fat
LAMB					
breast, lean, raw	**0**	0	179	0.0	11.2
breast, lean, roast	**0**	0	273	0.0	18.5
breast, raw	**0**	0	287	0.0	24.7
breast, roast	**0**	0	359	0.0	29.9
chop, with fat	**0**	0	277	0.0	23.0
cutlets, lean, grilled	**0**	0	238	0.0	13.8
cutlets, lean, barbecued	**0**	0	236	0.0	13.9
cutlets, barbecued	**0**	0	342	0.0	27.2
cutlets, grilled	**0**	0	367	0.0	29.9
ground, raw	**0**	0	196	0.0	13.3
ground, stewed	**0**	0	208	0.0	12.3
kebab, grilled	**0**	0	288	0.0	19.3
lean, raw	**0**	0	153	0.0	8.0
leg, lean, braised	**0**	0	204	0.0	10.5
leg, lean, roast	**0**	0	203	0.0	9.4
loin chop, grilled	**0**	0	277	0.0	22.1
loin chop, grilled, lean	**0**	0	213	0.0	10.7
shoulder, lean, roast	**0**	0	235	0.0	13.5
stewing, stewed	**0**	0	240	0.0	14.8

	GL	GI	Calories	Carbs	Fat
LEMON SOLE					
grilled	0	0	97	0.0	1.7
raw	0	0	83	0.0	1.5
steamed	0	0	91	0.0	0.9
LIVER					
calf, fried	0	0	188	0.0	9.6
chicken, fried	0	0	169	0.0	8.9
lamb, fried	0	0	237	0.0	12.9
pig, stewed	0	0	189	3.6	8.1
LIVER PÂTÉ					
reduced-fat	0	0	191	3.0	12.0
regular	0	0	348	0.8	32.7
LOBSTER					
boiled	0	0	103	0.0	1.6
MACKEREL					
fried	0	0	272	0.0	19.5
grilled	0	0	239	0.0	17.3
canned, in brine	0	0	237	0.0	17.9
canned, in olive oil	0	0	298	1.0	24.4

	GL	GI	Calories	Carbs	Fat
MACKEREL (CONTINUED)					
peppered	**0**	0	310	0.3	25.2
raw	**0**	0	220	0.0	16.1
smoked	**0**	0	354	0.0	30.9
MARLIN					
chargrilled	**0**	0	153	0.8	6.1
raw	**0**	0	99	0.0	0.2
smoked	**0**	0	120	0.0	0.1
MONKFISH					
grilled	**0**	0	96	0.0	0.6
raw	**0**	0	66	0.0	0.4
MULLET					
grilled	**0**	0	150	0.0	5.2
raw	**0**	0	115	0.0	4.0
MUSSELS					
boiled, no shells	**0**	0	28	3.5	2.7
boiled, with shells	**0**	0	28	0.9	0.7
raw	**0**	0	74	2.5	2.8

	GL	GI	Calories	Carbs	Fat

OCTOPUS

raw	**0**	0	83	trace	1.3

OMELETTE

cheese	**0**	0	271	trace	23.0
plain	**0**	0	195	0.0	16.8

OYSTERS

raw	**0**	0	65	2.7	1.3

PHEASANT

roasted	**0**	0	220	0.0	3.2

POLLACK

raw	**0**	0	82	0.0	1.0
steamed	**0**	0	82	0.0	1.3

PORK

chop, raw	**0**	0	257	0.0	18.2
chop, roasted	**0**	0	301	0.0	19.3
diced, kebabs, lean, grilled	**0**	0	179	0.0	4.7
diced, kebabs, grilled	**0**	0	189	0.0	6.1
diced, raw	**0**	0	147	0.0	7.2

	GL	GI	Calories	Carbs	Fat
PORK (CONTINUED)					
diced, slow-cooked	0	0	173	0.0	6.0
diced, lean, baked	0	0	184	0.0	6.8
diced, lean, raw	0	0	122	0.0	4.0
diced, lean, slow-cooked	0	0	169	0.0	5.4
fillet, strips, stir-fried	0	0	182	0.0	5.9
leg, raw, lean & fat	0	0	213	0.0	15.2
leg, roasted lean	0	0	182	0.0	5.5
loin, chop, lean, grilled	0	0	184	0.0	6.4
loin, chop, raw	0	0	270	0.0	21.7
raw	0	0	128	0.0	4.0
sausages, fried	3	28	308	9.9	23.9
sausages, grilled	3	28	294	9.8	22.1
side, grilled	0	0	320	0.0	23.4
steak, grilled	0	0	198	0.0	7.6
steak, raw	0	0	169	0.0	9.4
PRAWNS					
peeled, boiled	0	0	99	0.0	0.9
raw	0	0	76	0.0	0.6

	GL	GI	Calories	Carbs	Fat
RABBIT					
raw	0	0	137	0.0	5.5
stewed	0	0	114	0.0	3.4
ROE					
cod	0	0	104	0.0	1.9
SALAMI					
standard fat	0	0	438	0.5	39.2
raw	0	0	180	0.0	11.0
grilled	0	0	215	0.0	13.1
SALMON					
pink, canned, in brine	0	0	153	0.0	7.8
smoked	0	0	142	0.0	4.5
steamed	0	0	194	0.0	11.9
SARDINES					
canned, in brine	0	0	172	0.0	9.5
canned, in oil	0	0	220	0.0	14.1
canned, in tomato sauce	0	0	162	1.4	9.9
raw	0	0	165	0.0	9.2
grilled	0	0	195	0.0	10.4

MEATS, CHICKEN, SEAFOOD AND EGGS

	GL	GI	Calories	Carbs	Fat
SCALLOPS					
steamed	**0**	0	118	3.4	1.1
SEAWEED					
Irish Moss, dried, raw	**0**	0	8	trace	0.2
Kombu, dried, raw	**0**	0	43	trace	1.6
Nori, dried, raw	**0**	0	136	trace	1.5
Wakame, dried, raw	**0**	0	71	trace	2.4
SHARK					
raw	**0**	0	102	0.0	1.1
SHISH KEBAB					
standard fat	**0**	0	206	0.0	10.0
SHRIMP					
boiled	**0**	0	117	trace	2.4
canned, in brine	**0**	0	94	0.0	1.2
frozen	**0**	0	73	0.0	0.8
SNAPPER					
red, fried	**0**	0	126	0.0	3.1
red, raw	**0**	0	90	0.0	1.3

	GL	GI	Calories	Carbs	Fat

SQUID

	GL	GI	Calories	Carbs	Fat
raw	0	0	70	1.2	1.7

SUSHI

raw	0	0	143	24.3	2.2

SWORDFISH

grilled	0	0	139	0.0	5.2
raw	0	0	109	0.0	4.1

TONGUE

cooked	0	0	201	trace	14.0

TROUT

Brown, fillet, raw	0	0	112	0.0	3.8
Brown, fillet, steamed	0	0	135	0.0	4.5
Rainbow, fillet, grilled	0	0	135	0.0	8.4
Rainbow, fillet, raw	0	0	125	0.0	5.2
smoked	0	0	139	0.3	5.2

TUNA

canned, in brine	0	0	99	0.0	0.6
canned, in oil	0	0	189	0.0	9.0

	GL	GI	Calories	Carbs	Fat
TUNA (CONTINUED)					
canned, in spring water	**0**	0	108	0.0	0.6
canned, in water	**0**	0	105	0.1	0.8
pâté	**0**	0	236	0.4	18.6
raw	**0**	0	136	0.0	4.6
TURKEY					
breast, grilled	**0**	0	155	0.0	1.7
raw, dark meat only	**0**	0	105	0.0	2.5
raw, light meat only	**0**	0	104	0.0	0.8
roast, meat & skin	**0**	0	171	0.0	6.5
strips, stir fried	**0**	0	164	0.0	4.5
VEAL					
raw	**0**	0	109	0.0	2.7
roasted	**0**	0	230	0.0	11.5
VENISON					
raw	**0**	0	103	0.0	2.2
roasted	**0**	0	165	0.0	2.5

Chapter Three

Fruits

Fruits are nature's candy. They have high GI scores because they're packed with sugar, but you're unlikely to eat enough of any one fruit to throw your blood sugar out of whack, so they're perfect for a low-GL diet. Try to vary the fruits you eat and have them for snacks or for a healthy dessert.

	GL	GI	Calories	Carbs	Fat
APPLE					
baked, no sugar	**4**	38	43	10.7	0.1
baked, with sugar	**8**	38	78	20.1	0.1
Braeburn	**3**	32	47	10.5	0.1
dried	**23**	38	238	60.1	0.5
fresh	**4**	38	47	10.5	0.1
juice, unsweetened	**4**	40	38	9.9	0.1
juice, unsweetened, clear	**5**	44	45	10.4	0.1
juice, unsweetened, cloudy	**4**	37	49	11.9	0.1
APRICOTS					
canned, in juice	**5**	64	34	8.4	0.1
dried	**13**	30	188	43.4	0.7
fresh	**4**	57	31	7.2	0.1
AVOCADO					
fresh	**0+**	1	190	1.9	19.3
BANANA					
average	**12**	52	95	23.2	0.3
overripe	**12**	52	95	23.2	0.3
underripe	**10**	42	95	23.2	0.3

	GL	GI	Calories	Carbs	Fat
BLACKBERRIES					
fresh	**2**	40	25	5.1	0.2
CANTALOUPE					
fresh	**3**	65	19	4.2	0.1
CHERRIES					
canned, in light syrup	**4**	22	71	18.5	trace
fresh	**3**	22	48	11.5	0.1
pie filling	**10**	48	82	21.5	trace
CRANBERRY					
juice	**8**	56	61	14.4	0.0
juice cocktail	**6**	56	48	11.5	0.1
CURRANTS					
dried	**43**	64	267	67.8	0.4
DATES					
dried	**70**	103	270	68.0	0.2

	GL	GI	Calories	Carbs	Fat
FIGS					
dried	**32**	61	227	52.9	1.6
dried, cooked without sugar	**18**	61	126	29.4	0.9
FRUIT COCKTAIL					
canned, in juice	**4**	55	57	7.2	trace
GRAPEFRUIT					
fresh	**2**	30	30	6.8	0.1
juice	**4**	48	33	8.3	0.1
GRAPES					
black	**8**	59	60	15.4	0.1
red	**8**	53	60	15.4	0.1
white	**8**	53	60	15.4	0.1
HONEYDEW MELON					
fresh	**4**	65	28	6.6	0.1
KIWI					
Australia	**6**	58	49	10.6	0.5
local	**6**	53	49	10.6	0.5
New Zealand	**5**	47	49	10.6	0.5

	GL	GI	Calories	Carbs	Fat

LEMON

fresh	**1**	42	19	3.2	0.3

LYCHEES

canned, in syrup, drained	**14**	79	68	17.7	trace

MANDARINS

canned, in juice	**3**	42	32	7.7	trace
canned, in syrup	**6**	42	52	13.4	trace

MANGO

fresh	**7**	51	57	14.1	0.2

NECTARINES

fresh	**4**	42	40	9.0	0.1

ORANGE

fresh	**4**	42	37	8.5	0.1
juice, unsweetened	**5**	53	36	8.8	0.1

PAPAYA

fresh	**6**	56	45	11.3	0.1

	GL	GI	Calories	Carbs	Fat
PAWPAW					
fresh	**5**	56	36	8.8	0.1
PEACHES					
canned, in heavy syrup	**8**	58	55	14.0	trace
canned, in juice	**4**	45	39	9.7	trace
canned, in light syrup	**8**	57	55	14.0	trace
fresh	**3**	42	33	7.6	0.1
PEARS					
canned, in juice	**4**	45	33	8.5	trace
fresh	**4**	38	40	10.0	0.1
PINEAPPLE					
canned, in juice	**6**	46	47	12.2	trace
juice, unsweetened	**5**	46	47	12.2	trace
fresh	**7**	66	41	10.1	0.2
PLUMS					
canned	**6**	39	59	15.5	trace
fresh	**2**	24	36	8.8	0.1

	GL	GI	Calories	Carbs	Fat
PRUNES					
fresh	11	29	141	38.4	0.5
stewed, no sugar	6	29	81	19.5	0.3
stewed, with sugar	7	29	103	25.5	0.2
RAISINS					
dried	44	64	272	69.3	0.4
golden, dried	38	56	275	69.4	0.4
RASPBERRIES					
fresh	2	40	25	4.6	0.3
RHUBARB					
fresh	0+	0	7	0.8	0.1
stewed, no sugar	0+	0	7	0.7	0.1
STRAWBERRIES					
fresh	2	40	27	6.0	0.1
TANGERINES					
fresh	3	42	35	8.0	0.1

	GL	GI	Calories	Carbs	Fat
TOMATO JUICE					
no added sugar	**0+**	8	14	3.0	trace
WATERMELON					
fresh	**5**	72	31	7.1	0.3

Chapter Four

Vegetables, Nuts, Legumes and Soy

Vegetables are full of good vitamins and nuts, soy and legumes like beans and lentils are an excellent source of protein. Most have low-GL values, so get as many veggies into your diet as you can. For a healthy approach to the menu, make hearty vegetable-packed salads a part of your meals and find ways to make main courses based on tofu and legumes.

	GL	GI	Calories	Carbs	Fat
ALFALFA					
raw	**0+**	1	24	0.4	0.7
ARTICHOKE					
canned	**0**	0	30	5.5	0.1
globe, boiled	**0**	0	18	2.7	0.2
globe, raw	**0+**	1	18	2.7	0.2
Jerusalem, boiled	**0**	0	41	10.6	0.1
ASPARAGUS					
boiled	**0+**	1	26	1.4	0.8
raw	**0+**	1	25	2.0	0.6
AVOCADO					
raw	**0+**	1	190	1.9	19.3
BAKED BEANS					
reduced sugar & salt	**6**	48	73	12.5	0.6
regular	**7**	48	84	15.3	0.6
BAMBOO SHOOTS					
canned, drained	**0**	0	11	0.7	0.2

	GL	GI	Calories	Carbs	Fat
BEAN SPROUTS					
raw	**0+**	1	31	4.0	0.5
stir-fried in oil	**0+**	1	72	2.5	6.1
BEETS					
raw	**5**	64	36	7.6	0.1
BLACK-EYED PEAS					
soaked, boiled	**8**	42	116	19.9	0.7
BOK CHOY					
raw	**0+**	1	12	1.4	0.2
BROCCOLI					
boiled	**0+**	1	24	1.1	0.8
raw	**0+**	1	33	1.8	0.9
BRUSSELS SPROUTS					
boiled	**0+**	1	35	3.5	1.3
raw	**0+**	1	42	4.1	1.4

	GL	GI	Calories	Carbs	Fat
CABBAGE					
boiled	**0+**	1	16	2.2	0.4
Chinese, raw	**0**	0	12	1.4	0.2
dried	**0**	0	237	38.0	3.6
raw	**0+**	1	26	4.1	0.4
red, boiled	**0**	0	15	2.3	0.3
red, raw	**0**	0	21	3.7	0.3
Savoy, boiled	**0**	0	17	2.2	0.5
Savoy, raw	**0**	0	27	3.9	0.5
CARROTS					
raw	**4**	49	35	7.9	0.3
CASHEWS					
plain	**4**	22	573	18.1	48.2
roasted & salted	**4**	22	611	18.8	50.9
CASSAVA					
boiled	**15**	46	130	33.5	0.2
CAULIFLOWER					
boiled	**0**	0	28	2.1	0.9
raw	**0+**	1	34	3.0	0.9

	GL	GI	Calories	Carbs	Fat
CELERY					
boiled	**0**	0	8	0.8	0.3
raw	**0**	0	7	0.9	0.2
CHARD					
Swiss, boiled	**0**	0	20	3.2	0.1
Swiss, raw	**0**	0	19	2.9	0.2
CHICKPEAS					
canned	**7**	42	115	16.1	2.9
dried, boiled	**5**	28	121	18.2	2.1
CHICORY					
boiled	**0**	0	7	2.1	0.3
raw	**0**	0	11	2.8	0.6
CHILIES					
raw	**0**	0	26	4.2	0.3
CUCUMBER					
raw	**0+**	1	10	1.5	0.1

	GL	GI	Calories	Carbs	Fat
EGGPLANT					
fried	**0+**	1	190	2.8	31.9
raw	**0+**	1	15	2.2	0.4
ENDIVE					
raw	**0**	0	13	1.0	0.6
FAVA BEANS					
raw	**6**	79	59	7.2	1.0
FENNEL					
boiled	**0+**	1	11	1.5	0.2
raw	**0+**	1	12	1.8	0.2
GARLIC					
puree	**0+**	1	380	16.9	38.6
raw	**0+**	1	98	16.2	0.6
GREEN BEANS					
boiled	**0+**	1	25	4.7	0.1
raw	**0+**	1	24	3.2	0.5

	GL	GI	Calories	Carbs	Fat
HARICOT VERTS					
canned, drained	**6**	38	94	15.7	0.5
dried, boiled	**6**	33	95	17.2	0.5
HUMMUS					
plain	**7**	6	187	11.6	12.6
KALE					
curly, boiled	**0+**	1	24	1.0	1.1
curly, raw	**0+**	1	33	1.4	1.6
KIDNEY BEANS					
canned, drained	**6**	36	100	17.8	0.6
dried, boiled	**5**	28	100	17.4	0.5
KOHLRABI					
boiled, salted water	**0**	0	18	3.1	0.2
raw	**0**	0	23	3.7	0.2
LEEKS					
boiled	**0+**	1	22	2.6	0.7
raw	**0+**	1	22	2.9	0.5

	GL	GI	Calories	Carbs	Fat
LENTILS					
green, canned	5	48	64	10.2	0.4
green, dried, boiled	5	30	105	16.9	0.7
red, dried, boiled	5	26	100	17.5	0.4
LETTUCE					
Bibb	0	0	12	1.2	0.6
Iceberg	0+	1	13	1.9	0.3
Romaine	0	0	16	1.7	0.6
LIMA BEANS					
canned	5	36	77	13.0	0.5
dried, cooked	6	31	103	18.4	0.6
MUNG BEANS					
dried, boiled	6	39	91	15.3	0.4
MUSHROOMS					
fried	0+	1	157	0.3	16.2
raw	0+	1	13	0.4	0.5

	GL	GI	Calories	Carbs	Fat
OKRA					
boiled	**0+**	1	28	2.7	0.7
fried	**0+**	1	269	4.4	26.1
raw	**0+**	1	31	13.0	1.0
ONIONS					
baked	**0**	0	103	22.3	0.6
fried	**0**	0	164	14.1	11.2
pickled	**0**	0	24	4.9	0.2
raw	**0**	0	36	7.9	0.2
PARSNIPS					
boiled	**12**	97	66	12.9	1.2
raw	**12**	97	64	12.5	1.1
PEANUTS					
dry roasted	**1**	14	880	10.3	49.8
plain	**2**	14	563	12.5	46.6
roasted & salted	**1**	14	602	7.1	53.0
PEAS					
Marrowfat, boiled	**5**	39	80	13.0	0.4

	GL	GI	Calories	Carbs	Fat
PECANS					
raw	**1**	10	689	5.8	70.1
PEPPERS					
chili	**0+**	1	20	0.7	0.6
green bell, boiled	**0+**	1	18	2.6	0.5
green bell, raw	**0+**	1	15	2.6	0.3
red bell, boiled	**0+**	1	34	7.0	0.4
red bell, raw	**0+**	1	32	6.4	0.4
PINTO BEANS					
boiled	**7**	45	85	15.1	0.5
POTATOES					
baked	**27**	85	136	31.7	0.2
canned, drained, reheated	**10**	65	66	15.1	0.1
chips	**30**	57	530	53.3	34.2
French fries, microwaved	**24**	75	221	32.1	10.2
mashed	**13**	74	72	17.0	0.1
mashed, instant	12	86	57	13.5	0.1
peeled, boiled	**17**	101	72	17.0	0.1
unpeeled, boiled in skins	**13**	76	75	17.8	0.3

	GL	GI	Calories	Carbs	Fat
PUMPKIN					
boiled	**2**	75	13	2.1	0.3
raw	**2**	75	13	2.2	0.2
RADICCHIO					
raw	**0**	0	14	1.7	0.2
RADISHES					
raw	**0+**	1	12	1.9	0.2
RUTABAGA					
raw	**4**	72	24	5.0	0.3
SALAD GREENS					
raw	**0+**	1	17	2.0	0.2
SAUERKRAUT					
raw	**0**	0	9	1.1	trace
SEAWEED					
Irish Moss, dried, raw	**0**	0	8	trace	0.2
Kombu, dried, raw	**0**	0	43	trace	1.6
Nori, dried, raw	**0**	0	136	trace	1.5

	GL	GI	Calories	Carbs	Fat
SEAWEED (CONTINUED)					
Wakame, dried, raw	**0**	0	71	trace	2.4
raw	**0**	0	598	0.9	58.0
SHALLOTS					
pickled	**0**	0	77	18.0	0.1
raw	**0**	0	20	3.3	0.2
SOY BEANS					
cooked	**1**	20	141	5.1	7.3
SOY MILK					
plain	**1**	36	32	0.5	1.6
SOY YOGURT					
plain	**6**	50	72	12.9	1.8
SPINACH					
boiled	**0+**	1	19	0.8	0.8
raw	**0+**	1	25	1.6	0.8
SPLIT PEAS					
dried, cooked	**7**	32	126	22.7	0.9

	GL	GI	Calories	Carbs	Fat

SQUASH

	GL	GI	Calories	Carbs	Fat
boiled	0+	1	9	1.6	0.2
cooked, without sugar	0	0	4	1.0	0.0
raw	0+	1	12	2.2	0.2

SWEET CORN

	GL	GI	Calories	Carbs	Fat
baby, canned, drained	1	46	23	2.0	0.4
on cob, boiled	6	48	66	11.6	1.4

SWEET POTATOES

	GL	GI	Calories	Carbs	Fat
boiled	9	46	84	20.5	0.3

TOFU

	GL	GI	Calories	Carbs	Fat
fried	0+	1	261	2.0	17.7
steamed	0+	1	73	0.7	4.2

TOMATO

	GL	GI	Calories	Carbs	Fat
juice	0+	38	14	3.0	trace
raw	1	38	17	3.1	0.3

VEGEBURGER

	GL	GI	Calories	Carbs	Fat
grilled	5	59	196	8.0	11.1

	GL	GI	Calories	Carbs	Fat
WATERCRESS					
raw	**0+**	1	22	0.4	1.0
YAM					
boiled	**12**	37	133	33.0	0.3
ZUCCHINI					
boiled	**0+**	1	19	2.0	0.4
fried	**0+**	1	62	2.6	4.8
raw	**0+**	1	18	1.8	0.4

Chapter Five

Dairy, Cheeses,
Oils, Butter
and Alternatives

You'll get great calcium and protein from milk and cheese, and their low-GL vales mean they're great to eat in moderation. Buy a variety of cheese that you really like and keep it around for a treat. And when it comes to oil and butter, a little goes a long way toward tasty meals and a healthy GL score.

	GL	GI	Calories	Carbs	Fat
BUTTER					
reduced-fat	**0**	0	368	1.2	39.4
salted	**0**	0	744	0.6	82.2
spreadable	**0**	0	745	trace	82.5
unsalted	**0**	0	744	0.6	82.2
CHEESE					
Brie	**0**	0	343	0.0	29.1
Camembert	**0**	0	290	0.0	22.7
cheddar	**0**	0	416	0.1	32.7
cheddar, low-fat	**0**	0	273	0.0	15.8
cheddar, vegetarian	**0**	0	390	0.0	32.0
cream	**0**	0	439	0.0	47.5
Danish blue	**0**	0	342	0.0	28.9
double Gloucester	**0**	0	411	0.1	34.5
Edam	**0**	0	341	0.0	24.5
Edam, reduced-fat	**0**	0	229	0.0	10.9
Emmental	**0**	0	364	trace	28.0
feta	**0**	0	250	1.5	20.2
goat	**0**	0	320	1.0	25.8
Gouda	**0**	0	377	0.0	30.6
Halloumi	**0**	0	316	1.6	24.7

	GL	GI	Calories	Carbs	Fat
CHEESE (CONTINUED)					
Jarlsberg	0	0	362	0.0	28.0
mascarpone	0	0	437	4.1	43.6
mozzarella	0	0	257	0.0	20.3
Parmigiano Reggiano	0	0	384	0.0	28.0
Parmesan	0	0	415	0.9	29.7
ricotta	0	0	134	2.0	10.0
smoked, processed	0	0	303	0.2	24.5
Stilton	0	0	410	0.1	34.0
Taleggio	0	0	297	0.0	25.0
COCOA BUTTER					
regular	0	0	896	0.0	99.5
COTTAGE CHEESE					
low-fat	0	0	79	3.3	1.5
regular	0	0	101	3.1	3.0
DRIPPINGS					
beef	0	0	891	trace	99.0
GHEE					
regular	0	0	895	0.0	99.4

	GL	GI	Calories	Carbs	Fat
GROUND NUT OIL					
regular	0	0	824	0.0	91.6
ICE CREAM					
chocolate, 15% fat	6	37	215	16.8	15.1
full-fat	12	61	177	19.8	8.6
low-fat	7	50	119	13.7	6.0
LARD					
regular	0	0	891	0.0	99.9
MARGARINE					
regular	0	0	718	1.0	81.6
MILK					
condensed	34	61	333	55.5	10.1
low-fat	1	32	46	4.7	1.7
meal replacement drink	5	41	92	11.9	1.5
skim	1	32	32	4.4	0.3
soy	1	36	32	0.5	1.6
whole	1	31	66	4.5	3.9

	GL	GI	Calories	Carbs	Fat

OIL

	GL	GI	Calories	Carbs	Fat
canola	0	0	899	0.0	99.9
coconut	0	0	899	0.0	99.9
corn	0	0	899	0.0	99.9
olive	0	0	899	0.0	99.9
palm	0	0	899	0.0	99.9
peanut	0	0	899	0.0	99.9
sesame	0	0	899	0.0	99.7
soy	0	0	899	0.0	99.9
spray	0	0	498	0.0	55.2
sunflower	0	0	899	0.0	99.9
vegetable	0	0	899	0.0	99.9
walnut	0	0	899	0.0	99.9

YOGURT

	GL	GI	Calories	Carbs	Fat
drink	4	31	62	13.1	trace
fat-free, plain	2	20	54	8.2	0.2
low-fat	4	33	56	7.4	1.0
low-fat, fruit	4	31	78	13.7	1.1
low-fat, with sugar	2	33	56	7.4	1.0
probiotic drink	7	46	87	16.0	0.9
soy	6	50	72	12.9	1.8

Chapter Six

Desserts, Sweets and Snacks

Most of everyone's favorite treats are chock-full of sugar, which means their GL-values are through the roof. That doesn't mean you can never have chocolate or ice cream again— just make sure that your normal between-meal snacks are things like sweet and refreshing fruits or your favorite crunchy veggies. Save the sweets for special occasions.

	GL	GI	Calories	Carbs	Fat
BERRY MOUSSE					
low-fat	**4**	36	101	11.1	1.5
CAKE					
banana	**24**	51	257	46.9	7.4
sponge	**24**	46	467	52.4	27.2
vanilla-iced	**22**	42	490	52.4	30.6
CASHEWS					
plain	**4**	22	573	18.1	48.2
roasted & salted	**4**	22	611	18.8	50.9
CEREAL BAR					
plain	**47**	72	419	64.7	16.4
CHOCOLATE					
candy bar, caramel & cookie	**30**	44	492	68.5	26.1
candy bar, caramel-filled	**48**	62	473	77.3	18.9
candy bar, covered nuts	**23**	41	497	55.8	27.8
candy bar, milk	**33**	44	445	74.8	15.8
covered peanuts	**20**	33	520	60.2	28.7
instant pudding	**7**	47	111	14.8	6.3
milk	**28**	49	520	56.9	30.7

	GL	GI	Calories	Carbs	Fat
CHOCOLATE (CONTINUED)					
mousse	**6**	31	149	19.9	6.5
mousse, low-fat	**7**	37	123	18.0	3.7
plain	**26**	41	510	63.5	28.0
white	**26**	44	529	58.3	30.9
CHOCOLATE MOUSSE					
full-fat	**6**	31	149	19.9	6.5
low-fat	**7**	37	123	18.0	3.7
COFFEE					
black	**49**	79	454	62.2	21.8
COOKIES					
wafer	**51**	77	537	66.0	30.1
CORN CHIPS					
regular	**23**	42	459	54.3	31.9
CRACKERS					
gluten-free	**50**	87	480	58.0	23.0
table water	**54**	71	440	75.8	12.5

	GL	GI	Calories	Carbs	Fat
CREAM CRACKERS					
regular	**7**	65	444	10.0	14.5
EGG CUSTARD					
baked	**4**	35	118	11.0	6.0
FRUIT BARS					
baked	**67**	90	32	74.0	no fig
GLUTEN-FREE COOKIES					
regular	**42**	58	461	72.0	17.0
GRAHAM CRACKER					
plain	**40**	59	465	68.6	20.3
GRANOLA BAR					
plain	**30**	61	570	64.3	10.1
ICE CREAM					
full-fat	**12**	61	177	19.8	8.6
low-fat	**7**	50	119	13.7	6.0

	GL	GI	Calories	Carbs	Fat
JELLO					
fruit, sugar-free	0	0	6	0.1	0.0
JELLY BEANS					
regular	70	78	370	90.3	0.4
MARSHMALLOWS					
regular	51	62	327	83.1	0.0
NOUGAT					
regular	25	32	384	77.3	8.5
OATCAKES					
plain	34	54	412	63.0	15.1
OLIVES					
canned, in brine	0	0	103	0.0	11.0
PEANUTS					
dry-roasted	1	14	589	10.3	49.8
plain	2	14	563	12.5	46.6
roasted & salted	1	14	602	7.1	53.0

	GL	GI	Calories	Carbs	Fat
PECANS					
raw	**1**	10	689	5.8	70.1
PEPPERMINTS					
regular	**72**	70	393	102.7	0.7
POPCORN					
microwave	**32**	51	440	62.5	17.7
plain	**27**	55	593	48.7	42.8
PORK RINDS					
regular	**0**	0	606	0.2	46.0
POTATO CHIPS					
plain	**29**	54	530	53.3	34.2
PRETZELS					
plain	**66**	83	381	79.2	3.5
RICE CAKES					
plain	**66**	82	374	81.1	3.6

	GL	GI	Calories	Carbs	Fat
SESAME SEEDS					
raw	**0**	0	598	0.9	58.0
SHORTBREAD					
plain	**40**	64	509	63.3	27.5
SORBET					
fruit	**12**	50	97	24.8	0.3
TEA COOKIE					
plain	**41**	55	427	74.8	13.3
YOGURT					
drink	**4**	31	62	13.1	trace
fat-free	**2**	20	54	8.2	0.2
low-fat, with sugar	**2**	33	56	7.4	1.0
probiotic drink	**7**	46	87	16.0	0.9

Chapter Seven

Condiments, Spices, Sugar and Sweeteners

When you want to add extra excitement to your low-GL meals, turn to the spice rack. Most sugars and condiments have high-GL values and lots of calories, so you should use them sparingly, but herbs and spices have zero GL and virtually no calories. Try a few new flavors to transform your low-GL vegetables and whole grain dishes into more enticing entrees.

	GL	GI	Calories	Carbs	Fat
ALLSPICE					
ground	**0**	0	no fig	no fig	8.7
ANISE SEEDS					
whole	**0**	0	no fig	no fig	15.9
APPLESAUCE					
plain	**6**	38	64	16.7	0.1
ASPARTAME					
regular	**0**	0	392	95.0	0.0
BAKING POWDER					
regular	**0**	0	157	37.8	0.0
BASIL					
dried	**0**	0	251	43.2	4.0
fresh	**0**	0	40	5.1	0.8
BAY LEAF					
dried	**0**	0	313	48.6	8.4

	GL	GI	Calories	Carbs	Fat
CARAWAY SEEDS					
whole	0	0	no fig	no fig	14.6
CAYENNE					
ground	0	0	318	31.7	17.3
CHERVIL					
dried	0	0	237	37.8	3.9
CHILI POWDER					
ground	0	0	0	unknown	16.8
CHINESE 5 SPICE					
ground	0	0	0	unknown	8.7
CHIVES					
fresh	0	0	20	1.7	0.0
CHOCOLATE-NUT SPREAD					
regular	20	33	549	60.5	33.0
CINNAMON					
ground	0	0	261	55.5	3.2

	GL	GI	Calories	Carbs	Fat
CLOVES					
dried	**0**	0	no fig	no fig	20.1
CORIANDER					
leaves, dried	**0**	0	279	41.7	4.8
leaves, fresh	**0**	0	20	1.8	0.6
seeds	**0**	0	no fig	no fig	17.8
CREAM-BASED DIP					
regular	**0**	0	360	4.0	37.0
CUMIN					
seeds	**0**	0	no fig	no fig	18.2
CURRY					
powder	**0**	0	233	26.1	10.8
DILL					
dried	**0**	0	253	42.2	4.4
fresh	**0**	0	25	0.9	0.8
seeds	**0**	0	no fig	no fig	14.5

	GL	GI	Calories	Carbs	Fat
FENNEL					
seeds	0	0	no fig	no fig	14.9
FENUGREEK					
leaves, fresh	0	0	35	4.8	0.2
seeds	0	0	no fig	no fig	7.4
FRUCTOSE					
regular	0	19	374	100.0	0.0
GARAM MASALA					
ground	0	0	379	45.2	15.1
GARLIC					
powder	0	0	310	12.7	1.7
GELATIN					
regular	0	0	338	0.0	0.0
GINGER					
fresh	0	0	49	9.5	0.7
ground	0	0	258	60.0	3.3

CONDIMENTS, SPICES, SUGAR AND SWEETENERS

	GL	GI	Calories	Carbs	Fat
GLUCOSE					
regular	**100**	100	375	100.0	0.0
HERBS					
dried	**0+**	1	181	36.3	8.5
fresh	**0+**	1	34	2.7	1.3
HUMMUS					
plain	**7**	6	187	11.6	12.6
LEMON JUICE					
fresh	**1**	42	7	1.6	trace
LICORICE					
powder	**0**	0	no fig	no fig	1.7
MACE					
ground	**0**	0	no fig	no fig	32.4
MARJORAM					
dried	**0**	0	271	42.5	7.0

	GL	GI	Calories	Carbs	Fat

MAYONNAISE

regular	**0**	0	691	1.7	75.6

MINT

dried	**0**	0	279	34.6	4.6
fresh	**0+**	1	43	5.3	0.7

MIXED HERBS

dried	**0**	0	261	36.3	8.5

MUSTARD

ground	**0**	0	452	20.7	45.1
whole grain	**0+**	1	140	4.2	10.2

NUTMEG

ground	**0**	0	0	unknown	36.3

OREGANO

dried	**0**	0	306	49.5	10.3
fresh	**0**	0	66	9.7	2.0

PAPRIKA

ground	**0**	0	289	34.9	13.0

CONDIMENTS, SPICES, SUGAR AND SWEETENERS

	GL	GI	Calories	Carbs	Fat
PARSLEY					
dried	**0**	0	181	14.5	7.0
fresh	**0+**	1	34	2.7	1.3
PEANUT BUTTER					
regular	**30**	23	606	13.1	51.8
PEPPER					
black	**0**	0	0	unknown	3.3
white	**0**	0	0	unknown	2.1
POPPY SEEDS					
whole	**0**	0	no fig	no fig	44.0
ROSEMARY					
dried	**0**	0	331	46.4	15.2
fresh	**0**	0	99	13.5	4.4
SAFFRON					
regular	**0**	0	310	61.5	5.9

	GL	GI	Calories	Carbs	Fat
SAGE					
dried	**0**	0	315	42.7	12.7
fresh	**0**	0	119	15.6	4.6
SALT					
reduced-sodium	**0**	0	0	0.0	0.0
regular	**0**	0	0	0.0	0.0
SOY SAUCE					
regular	**0+**	1	43	8.2	trace
STOCK					
cube, beef	**0**	0	179	3.2	0.6
cube, chicken	**0+**	1	237	9.9	15.4
cube, vegetable	**0+**	1	253	11.6	17.3
homemade, chicken	**0**	0	16	0.1	0.1
STUFFING					
sage & onion	**21**	74	269	29.0	15.1

	GL	GI	Calories	Carbs	Fat
SUCROSE					
regular	**68**	68	394	100.0	0.0
SYRUP					
corn	**50**	63	298	79.0	0.0
maple	**36**	54	262	67.2	0.2
TAMARIND					
leaves, fresh	**0**	0	115	18.2	2.1
TARRAGON					
dried	**0**	0	295	42.8	7.2
fresh	**0**	0	49	6.3	1.1
THYME					
dried	**0**	0	276	45.3	7.4
fresh	**0**	0	95	15.1	2.5
TURMERIC					
ground	**0**	0	no fig	no fig	7.0

	GL	GI	Calories	Carbs	Fat
VINEGAR					
balsamic	**0**	0	3	0.6	0.0
regular	**0**	0	22	0.6	0.0
white wine	**0**	0	21	0.3	0.0
WORCHESTERSHIRE SAUCE					
regular	**0+**	1	65	15.5	0.1

CONDIMENTS, SPICES, SUGAR AND SWEETENERS

Chapter Eight

Soups, Sandwiches and Prepared Foods

When you don't have time to cook a proper low-GL meal, it's all too easy to opt for a quick-and-easy but also diet-busting food. However, if you choose wisely, there are some easy alternatives like whole-grain pizzas and soups that will make sure your night out of the kitchen keeps your diet right on track.

	GL	GI	Calories	Carbs	Fat
CHOCOLATE-NUT SPREAD					
regular	**20**	33	549	60.5	33.0
HONEY					
manuka	**31**	39	314	80.0	0.0
regular	**42**	55	288	76.4	0.0
HUMMUS					
plain	**1**	6	187	11.6	12.6
JAM					
apricot, reduced-sugar	**17**	55	123	31.9	0.1
strawberry	**39**	56	261	69.0	0.0
MACARONI & CHEESE					
regular	**6**	47	86	12.0	2.7
MARMALADE					
orange	**33**	48	261	69.5	0.0
OMELETTE					
plain	**0**	0	195	0.0	16.8

	GL	GI	Calories	Carbs	Fat
OYSTERS					
raw	**0**	0	65	2.7	1.3
PÂTÉ					
liver	**0**	0	348	0.8	32.7
tuna	**0**	0	236	0.4	18.6
vegetable	**0**	0	173	5.9	13.4
PEANUT BUTTER					
regular	**3**	23	606	13.1	51.8
PIZZA					
cheese & tomato, pan	**13**	36	249	35.1	7.5
cheese & tomato, thin crust	**11**	36	238	30.1	8.8
cheese, thin crust	**10**	30	277	33.9	10.3
vegetarian	**14**	49	216	29.6	6.9
RAVIOLI					
meat-filled	**3**	39	75	7.0	0.5

	GL	GI	Calories	Carbs	Fat
SOUP					
lentil, canned	**3**	44	39	6.5	0.2
minestrone, canned	**2**	39	31	5.7	0.5
pea	**5**	66	40	7.3	0.8
tomato, canned	**2**	38	52	5.9	3.0

Chapter Nine

Drinks

Most beverages are diet disasters in disguise. The best
approach is to drink more water, which has zero GL and
zero calories. Treat flavored drinks like candy and sweets.
Drink water to stay hydrated the same way you eat healthy
food to stay full, and make juice and soda a special treat
instead of a part of every meal.

	GL	GI	Calories	Carbs	Fat

APPLE JUICE

	GL	GI	Calories	Carbs	Fat
unsweetened	4	40	38	9.9	0.1
unsweetened, clear	5	44	45	10.4	0.1
unsweetened, cloudy	4	37	49	11.9	0.1

BEER

amber ale	1	110	30	trace	trace
lager	1	110	29	trace	trace
lager, alcohol-free	2	110	7	1.5	trace
lager, low-alcohol	2	110	10	1.5	trace
pale ale	2	110	30	2.2	trace
stout	2	110	30	1.5	trace

BRANDY

standard	0	0	222	trace	0.0

CAPPUCCINO

unsweetened	1	31	66	4.5	3.9

CIDER

dry	3	110	36	2.6	0.0
low-alcohol	4	110	17	3.6	0.0
sweet	5	110	42	4.3	0.0

	GL	GI	Calories	Carbs	Fat
COFFEE					
black, no sugar	**0**	0	0	4.5	0.0
CRANBERRY JUICE					
regular	**7**	52	61	14.4	0.0
CRANBERRY JUICE COCKTAIL					
regular	**6**	56	48	11.5	0.1
GIN					
standard	**0**	0	222	trace	0.0
GRAPEFRUIT JUICE					
unsweetened	**4**	48	33	8.3	0.1
HERBAL TEA					
unsweetened	**0**	0	0	0.2	0.0
HOT CHOCOLATE					
made with water	**2**	51	78	4.0	2.4
LEMONADE					
low-calorie	**0**	0	0	0.1	0.0

	GL	GI	Calories	Carbs	Fat

MILK SHAKE

| chocolate, low-fat | **5** | 41 | 69 | 11.3 | 1.6 |

NUTRIENT-FORTIFIED DRINK

| plain | **5** | 41 | 98 | 11.7 | 3.6 |

ORANGE JUICE

| unsweetened | **5** | 53 | 36 | 8.8 | 0.1 |

PINEAPPLE JUICE

| unsweetened | **5** | 46 | 41 | 10.5 | 0.1 |

RUM

| standard | **0** | 0 | 222 | trace | 0.0 |

SHERRY

| dry | **0** | 0 | 116 | 1.4 | 0.0 |

SMOOTHIE

| raspberry | **4** | 33 | 53 | 11.9 | trace |

	GL	GI	Calories	Carbs	Fat
SODA					
diet	**0**	0	0	0.0	0.0
regular	**6**	53	41	10.9	0.0
SOY MILK					
chocolate	**3**	34	71	10.0	1.7
SPORTS DRINK					
regular	**3**	43	29	6.9	trace
TEA					
black	**0**	0	0	trace	trace
chamomile	**0**	0	1	0.2	trace
Chinese	**0**	0	1	0.2	0.0
decaffeinated	**0**	0	1	0.2	0.0
herbal	**0**	0	1	0.2	trace
Indian	**0**	0	trace	trace	trace
TOMATO JUICE					
no added sugar	**0+**	8	14	3.0	trace
VERMOUTH					
dry	**0**	0	109	3.0	0.0

	GL	GI	Calories	Carbs	Fat
VODKA					
standard	**0**	0	222	trace	0.0
WATER					
flat	**0**	0	0	0.0	0.0
seltzer	**0**	0	0	0.0	0.0
WHISKEY					
standard	**0**	0	222	trace	0.0
WINE					
red	**0**	0	68	0.2	0.0
white	**0**	0	66	0.6	0.0

Other Ulysses Press Books

The Easy GL Diet Handbook: Lose Weight with the Revolutionary Glycemic Load Program
Dr. Fedon Alexander Lindberg, **$10.00**

Using these more accurate and sensible GL scores, *The Easy GL Diet Handbook* offers a plan for healthy weight loss and reduced risk of diabetes that's easier to follow. It also includes numerous foods that the Atkins, South Beach and GI diets wrongly consider "off-limits."

The GL Cookbook and Diet Plan: A Glycemic Load Weight-Loss Program with Over 150 Delicious Recipes
Nigel Denby, **$12.95**

Offers a vast selection of GL-scored recipes so dieters can choose dishes they love while following a proven program for permanent weight loss without hunger.

The Leptin Boost Diet: Unleash Your Fat-Controlling Hormones for Maximum Weight Loss
Scott Isaacs, M.D., **$14.95**

A series of recent medical breakthroughs have confirmed what physicians suspected all along—obesity is a hormonal disorder. *The Leptin Boost Diet* transforms these findings into a unique and easy-to-follow weight-loss program that is perfect for people whose out-of-balance hormones make it impossible to lose weight on other diets.

Mastering Cortisol: Stop Your Body's Stress Hormone from Making You Fat around the Middle
Marilyn Glenville, **$15.95**

Details specific ways to counter cortisol with a tailor-made exercise plan that will slim the belly. Based on breakthrough genetic tests, the program also recommends specific vitamins and minerals and explains which foods will work best for the reader.

The pH Balance Diet: Restore Your Acid-Alkaline Levels to Eliminate Toxins and Lose Weight
Bharti Vyas & Suzanne Le Quesne, **$12.95**

Tells how to pH-test one's body, correct imbalances, and eliminate toxic overload by following a dietary way of life that works. An easy-to-follow section with over 40 recipes is included to help guide readers through the plan.

The Simple 0-to-10 GI Diet: Lose Weight with the Easy Food-Scoring System Based on the Glycemic Index
Azmina Govindji & Nina Puddefoot, **$12.95**

By simplifying the scoring system and creating an easy-to-follow plan, this handbook offers a no-hassle program to lose weight and maintain a healthy long-term diet.

To order these books: call 800-377-2542 or 510-601-8301, fax 510-601-8307, e-mail ulysses@ulyssespress.com, or write to Ulysses Press, P.O. Box 3440, Berkeley, CA 94703. All retail orders are shipped free of charge. California residents must include sales tax. Allow two to three weeks for delivery.